My Medical Manager

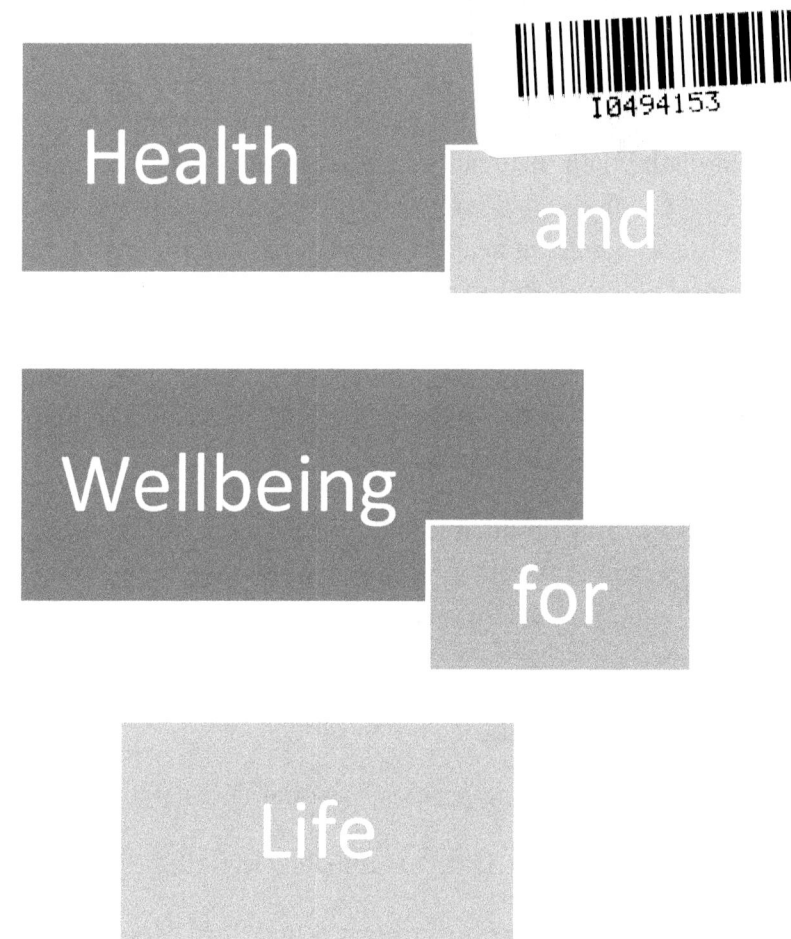

Health and Wellbeing for Life

My Medical Manager

For additional copies

https://www.createspace.com/4749039

Welcome to **"My Medical Manager"**, this convenient, easy to use booklet is designed to assist in caring for a person's medical needs and the needs of their family members. It will help keep all things MEDICAL in order.

It has always been said that patients have a responsibility to keep a record with their medications and allergies, a list of chronic illnesses, special conditions, surgeries, treatments, etc... as these records could be crucial to helping health care workers save lives. The Surgeon General writes on-going reports regarding the importance of creating a "Personal Health History", AARP writes newsletters and stories of the need of a "Personal Medical History". Both give a summary of what should be written and provide links to create a shortened version of a medical history.

People are more productive and proactive if a step-by-step guide is given to them to fill out as opposed to "writing it on a piece of paper", in a "journal" or on a website (which is inconvenient when an emergency strikes).

My Medical Manager is perfect for:

*Daily use   *Emergencies / Natural Disasters

*Out of state/country family members *Traveling/Vacation/holiday

*Home Health Agencies, Caregivers and Providers

It's simple.......

Each and every day, situations and emergencies happen. Although we cannot control what happens to us, we can control how we handle them and how **BEING PREPARED** will greatly assist all professionals and specialists that are there to help. For health and safety, be prepared and take responsibility.

Welcome to **My Medical Manager,** a Guide to all things YOU. This easy to fill booklet is designed to assist you in caring for your medical needs and the needs of family members. All too often, if an emergency strikes, people are caught unprepared. This convenient booklet allows you to keep your information and documents in order and easy to reach. Keep one for each member of your family. Perfect for daily use, emergencies, out-of state/country family members and while traveling or on vacation. **Keep Yourself Prepared**.

BRING BOOKLET WITH YOU TO ALL APPOINTMENTS.

- Identification Sheet – This form lists your name, date of birth, address, telephone number, insurance, and policy number, and allergy summary.

- Medication, Vitamins, Supplements Record – A list of medicines prescribed or given to you, Vitamins, Supplements and Over the Counter medications, including doses and schedules. Pharmacy names, locations and phone numbers.

- Chronic Conditions – A list of significant illnesses, allergies and alerts. (ex: Diabetes, high blood pressure, heart disease, stroke, food, drugs, animal, seasonal, medical alert ID, etc…)

- History– A brief description of any significant family history of disease and your health habits.

- Physicians – Names, Locations and Phone Numbers of ALL treating personnel.

- Surgeries, Treatments, Procedures and Locations – Information regarding Hospitalizations, Surgeries,

Treatments, Therapies, Clinical Treatment, and Social Work

- Imaging, X-ray, and Lab Studies, Screenings Performed: – Name of study, date, location and phone number of x-rays, mammograms, ultrasounds, CT scans, additional scans, lab work (common examples include: throat culture, urinalysis, cholesterol level, and complete blood count (CBC)and Blood Type - **Blood typing is not part of routine lab work.**

- Immunization Record – A form documenting immunizations given for disease such as polio, measles, mumps, rubella, and the flu. Parents should maintain a copy of their children's immunization records with other important papers.

- Hospital, Out-Patient, Therapy location preferences.

- Consent and Authorization Forms, Living Will, Power of Attorney, DNR, Guardian, Funeral, Organ Donor forms – Copies of consents for admission, treatment, surgery, and release of information. (**Some forms MAY BE State specific, contact your State via their website or your local library for State Specific Forms)

- Personal / Historical Information

- Memorialization Information

- Health, Life, Major Medical, Home, Automotive Insurance Information

One note of caution: *Never put a social security number on this list.* **It's not important for responders and if the list is lost, there is already a birthdate and name on each page.**

Name:

_____

_____

Male_____ Female_____	Race:	Religion:

Spouse / Other:

_____

_____

Address:

_____

_____

Telephone Number:

_____

_____

Date of Birth:

_____

In Case of Emergency (Name and Phone Number):

_____

_____

Primary Care Physician:

_____

_____

Allergies: (SUMMARY – Brief Description)

_____

_____

Insurance: (attach copy of card and/or print information)

_____

Medication, Vitamins, Supplements, Over the Counter Records

Medication	Dosage Amount	Schedule	Pharmacy Name / Phone

Medication, Vitamins, Supplements Record

Pharmacy – Attach Medication Labels

Medication/Supplement/Vitamin	Medication/Supplement/Vitamin
Instruction:	Instruction:
Medication/Supplement/Vitamin	Medication/Supplement/Vitamin
Instruction:	Instruction:
Medication/Supplement/Vitamin	Medication/Supplement/Vitamin
Instruction:	Instruction:
Medication/Supplement/Vitamin	Medication/Supplement/Vitamin
Instruction:	Instruction:
Medication/Supplement/Vitamin	Medication/Supplement/Vitamin

PHARMACY: Use additional page or back of age if necessary

Medication, Vitamins, Supplements Record

Pharmacy – Attach Medication Labels

Medication/Supplement/Vitamin	Medication/Supplement/Vitamin
Instruction:	Instruction:
Medication/Supplement/Vitamin	Medication/Supplement/Vitamin
Instruction:	Instruction:
Medication/Supplement/Vitamin	Medication/Supplement/Vitamin
Instruction:	Instruction:
Medication/Supplement/Vitamin	Medication/Supplement/Vitamin
Instruction:	Instruction:
Medication/Supplement/Vitamin	Medication/Supplement/Vitamin

PHARMACY: Use additional page if necessary

Chronic Conditions / Illnesses / Allergies

List significant illnesses, allergies and alerts. (ex: Diabetes, high blood pressure, heart disease, stroke, food, drugs, animal, seasonal, medical alert ID, etc…)

ALLERGY	REACTION	TREATMENT

ILLNESS	DATE OF ONSET	TREATMENT

ALERTS	REASON	TREATMENT/NOTIFICATION

Additional Information

History

Significant personal and family history of disease and your health habits.

Have you ever had:

Scarlet Fever   YES   NO
Meningitis   YES   NO
Infectious Mononucleosis   YES   NO
Tuberculosis   YES   NO
Exposure to TB   YES   NO
Malaria   YES   NO
Bronchitis   YES   NO
Pneumonia   YES   NO
Pleurisy   YES   NO
Hepatitis (yellow jaundice)   YES   NO
Bladder infections   YES   NO
Rheumatic fever   YES   NO
Kidney disease   YES   NO
Hives   YES   NO
Hay fever/sinusitis   YES   NO

Asthma   YES   NO
Emphysema   YES   NO
Arthritis   YES   NO
Back trouble   YES   NO
High blood pressure   YES   NO
Heart disease   YES   NO
Anemia   YES   NO
Bleeding tendency   YES   NO
Nose bleeds   YES   NO
Ulcer   YES   NO
Cancer   YES   NO
Hemorrhoids   YES   NO
Blood transfusion   YES   NO
Diabetes   YES   NO

FAMILY HISTORY

Has any blood relative had any of the following, If yes, what relationship:

Anemia   YES   NO   Relationship:
Leukemia   YES   NO   Relationship:
Repeated infections   YES   NO   Relationship:
Crippling arthritis   YES   NO   Relationship:
Chronic lung disease   YES   NO   Relationship:
High blood pressure   YES   NO   Relationship:
Kidney disease   YES   NO   Relationship:
Asthma   YES   NO   Relationship:
Severe allergies   YES   NO   Relationship:
Mental illness   YES   NO   Relationship:
Convulsions or seizures   YES   NO   Relationship:
Migraine headaches   YES   NO   Relationship:
Diabetes   YES   NO   Relationship:
Gout   YES   NO   Relationship:
Obesity   YES   NO   Relationship:
Thyroid trouble   YES   NO   Relationship:
Peptic ulcer   YES   NO   Relationship:
Chronic diarrhea   YES   NO   Relationship:
Cancer   YES   NO   Relationship:
Suicide   YES   NO   Relationship:
Gallbladder Disease   YES   NO   Relationship
Alcoholism   YES   NO   Relationship:

OPERATIONS

C Section   YES   NO
Tonsils   YES   NO
Gall Blander   YES   NO
Breast   YES   NO
Uterus and/or Ovary   YES   NO
Prostate   YES   NO
Hernia   YES   NO

Thyroid   YES   NO
Varicose Veins   YES   NO
Hemorrhoids   YES   NO
Heart   YES   NO
Kidney Stones   YES   NO
Other   YES   NO

INJURIES

Head   YES   NO
Chest   YES   NO
Abdomen   YES   NO
Broken bones   YES   NO
Back   YES   NO
Other   YES   NO

ALLERGIES

Penicillin: YES   NO
Sulfa: YES   NO
Dye: YES   NO
Codeine: YES   NO
Cosmetics: YES   NO
Tetanus antitoxin: YES   NO

Foods: YES   NO
Please List:

Other drugs: YES   NO
Please List:

Seasonal: YES   NO
Please List:

IMMUNIZATIONS

Tetanus shot   YES   NO
Polio oral   YES   NO
Flu shot   YES   NO
Others (list)   YES   NO

GENERAL
Have you had any of these symptoms?

Tire easily weakness   YES   NO
Market weight change   YES   NO
Night sweats   YES   NO
Persistent fever   YES   NO
Sensitivity to heat   YES   NO
Sensitivity to cold   YES   NO
Hernia   YES   NO

History (continued)

Significant personal and family history of disease and your health habits.

SKIN
Eruptions (rash)   YES   NO

Change in color   YES   NO

Changes in hair   YES   NO

Changes in nails   YES   NO

EYES
Trouble seeing / Eye pain   YES   NO

Inflamed eyes   YES   NO

Double vision   YES   NO

Worn glasses   YES   NO

EARS
Loss of hearing   YES   NO

Ringing in ears   YES   NO

Discharge   YES   NO

MOUTH
Sore gums   YES   NO

Soreness of tongue   YES   NO

Dental problems   YES   NO

THROAT
Post nasal drainage   YES   NO

Soreness   YES   NO

Hoarseness   YES   NO

BREASTS
Lumps   YES   NO

Discharge   YES   NO

NOSE
Excess discharge   YES   NO

Nosebleeds   YES   NO

Loss of smell   YES   NO

Frequent colds   YES   NO

Obstruction   YES   NO

CARDIO-RESPIRATORY SYSTEM
Cough persisting   YES   NO

Sputum (phlegm)   YES   NO

Bloody sputum   YES   NO

Wheezing   YES   NO

Chest pain or discomfort   YES   NO

Pain on breathing   YES   NO

Shortness of breath   YES   NO

Difficult breathing lying down YES NO

Swelling of ankles   YES   NO

Bluish fingers or lips   YES   NO

High blood pressure   YES   NO

Palpitations   YES   NO

Vein trouble   YES   NO

Other   YES   NO   Please List:

GASTRO-INTESTINAL
Symptoms now or in the last six months?

Change in appetite   YES   NO

Difficulty swallowing   YES   NO

Heartburn   YES   NO

Abdominal distress   YES   NO

Belching or excess gas   YES   NO

Abdominal enlargement   YES   NO

Nausea   YES   NO

Vomiting   YES   NO

Vomiting of blood   YES   NO

Rectal bleeding   YES   NO

Tarry stools   YES   NO

Jaundice   YES   NO

Constipation   YES   NO

Hemorrhoids   YES   NO

Need for laxatives YES   NO

History (continued)

Significant personal and family history of disease and your health habits.

GENITOURINARY SYSTEM

Unable to hold urine   YES   NO
Pain or burning   YES   NO
Blood in urine   YES   NO
Lack of sex drive   YES   NO

Increase in urination frequency (day)   YES   NO
Increase in urination frequency (night)   YES   NO
Need to urinate without much urine   YES   NO
Smell / Discharge with urine   YES   NO

ENDOCRINE

Cortisone treatment   YES   NO
Diabetes   YES   NO

Thyroid trouble   YES   NO
Adrenal trouble   YES   NO

LOCOMOTOR

Swollen joints   YES   NO
Stiffness   YES   NO
Deformity of joints   YES   NO

Muscle cramps   YES   NO
Muscle weakness   YES   NO
Pain in joints   YES   NO

NERVOUS SYSTEM

Headache   YES   NO
Dizziness   YES   NO
Fainting   YES   NO
Convulsions or fits   YES   NO
Nervousness   YES   NO
Sleeplessness   YES   NO

Depression   YES   NO
Change in Sensation   YES   NO
Memory Loss   YES   NO
Poor Coordination   YES   NO
Weakness or paralysis of muscles   YES   NO

OBSTETRICS-GYNECOLOGY

Duration_____   Days_____
Flow: _____ Light_____ Normal_____ Heavy_____
Pain with periods: YES_____ NO_____
Duration: _____ Days_____
Started menstruating at age_____
Date of last period _____/_____/_____
Interval between periods_____

SOCIAL BEHAVIOR

Alcohol   YES   NO   Per Day_____   Per Week_____
Smoking   YES   NO   Per Day_____   Per Week_____
Recreational Drugs   YES   NO   Per Day_____   Per Week_____

Physicians / Therapists / Clinics

Names, Locations and Phone Numbers of ALL treating personnel.

PHYSICIAN NAME	SPECIALITY	PHONE NUMBER	LOCATION

Surgeries, Procedures, Treatments and Locations

Brief description of Hospitalizations, Surgeries, Treatments,
Therapies, Clinical Treatment, Social Work

TREATMENT/PROCEDURE	SPECIALIST	LOCATION	PHONE / CONTACT

Imaging, X-ray, and Lab Studies, Screenings Performed
Name of study, date, location and phone number

STUDY	DATE	LOCATION	PHONE / CONTACT

x-rays, mammograms, ultrasounds, CT scans, additional scans, lab work (common examples include: throat culture, urinalysis, cholesterol level, and complete blood count (CBC)and Blood Type – **Blood typing is not part of routine lab work.**

Immunization Record

Document immunizations given for disease such as polio, measles, mumps, rubella, the flu and tetanus. Parents should maintain a copy of their children's immunization records with other important papers.

IMMUNIZATION	DATE	SPECIALIST	PHONE / CONTACT

Immunization Record

Document immunizations given for disease such as polio, measles, mumps, rubella, the flu and tetanus. Parents should maintain a copy of their children's immunization records with other important papers.

IMMUNIZATION	DATE	SPECIALIST	PHONE / CONTACT

Hospital, Out-Patient, Therapy and Clinic preferences

Primary Location
Name / Type:

_____

Location:

_____

Contact / Phone Number:

_____

Location
Name / Type:

_____

Location:

_____

Contact / Phone Number:

_____

Location
Name / Type:

_____

Location:

_____

Contact / Phone Number:

_____

Location
Name / Type:

_____

Location:

_____

Contact / Phone Number:

_____

Consent, Authorization, Living Will, Power of Attorney, DNR, Guardian, Funeral, Organ Donor information/forms

Will / Living Will   YES   NO
Contact Name, Location, Phone Number:

_____

_____

Attorney / Guardian / Power of Attorney   YES   NO
Contact Name, Location, Phone Number:

_____

_____

DNR / Organ Donor   YES   NO
Contact Name, Location, Phone Number:

_____

_____

Persons to be Notified   YES   NO
Name:

_____

Relationship:

_____

Phone Number:

_____

Persons to be Notified   YES   NO
Name:

_____

Relationship:

_____

Phone Number:

_____

Personal / Historical Information
MILITARY STATISTICS

Branch of Service:	Service Serial Number:
Date Entered Service:	Location Entered:
Date of Separation:	Location Separation:
Grade, Rank or Rating:	Wars/Conflicts Served:

EDUCATION / OCCUPATION / VOLUNTEER

Location:

Years:

Degrees:

Honors:

Special Achievements / Recognitions:

Civic or Public Offices Held:

Occupation / Employer:

Volunteer / Charity / Location:

Organization(s):

MEMORIALIZATION INFORMATION

Location: (Cemetery or Other)

Address:

Telephone and Contact:

Type of Property:

Mausoleum   Ground Burial   Lawn Crypt
          Urn / Niche   **(circle one)**

Description:

Location of Deed:

Type of Memorial: Companion   Individual   **(circle one)**

Manufacturer:

Additional Remarks / Notes:

_____

_____

_____

_____

_____

_____

_____

_____

_____

Insurance Information

Health Insurance   YES   NO
Provider/Plan, ID#, Group Number, Phone Number:

_____

_____

_____

Secondary Insurance   YES   NO
Provider/Plan, ID#, Group Number, Phone Number:

_____

_____

_____

Major Medical Insurance   YES   NO
Provider/Plan, ID#, Group Number, Phone Number:

_____

_____

_____

Life Insurance   YES   NO

Provider/Plan, ID#, Group Number, Phone Number:

_____

_____

_____

Additional Insurance / Medical Benefits
YES   NO

Provider/Plan, ID#, Group Number, Phone Number:

_____

_____

_____

Additional Insurance / Benefits   YES   NO

Carrier/Plan, ID#, Group Number, Phone Number:

_____

_____

Additional Insurance Information

Home Owners Insurance   **YES**   **NO**

Carrier/Plan, ID#, Group Number, Phone Number:

_____

_____

_____

Flood Insurance   **YES**   **NO**

Carrier/Plan, ID#, Group Number, Phone Number:

_____

_____

_____

Automotive Insurance   **YES**   **NO**

Carrier/Plan, ID#, Group Number, Phone Number:

_____

_____

_____

Banking / Safe Deposit / Trusts   **YES**   **NO**

_____

_____

Additional Information

_____

_____

_____

_____

_____

_____

_____

_____

_____

_____

_____

_____

_____

_____

_____

_____

Additional Information

_____

_____

_____

_____

_____

_____

_____

Copies of consents for admission, treatment, surgery, and release of information notification: **Some forms MAY BE State specific, contact your State via their website or your local library for State Specific Forms**

My Medical Manager and its' creators, designers and authors make no health, medical, or diagnostic claims regarding the interpretation or utilization of any information contained herein and/or recorded by the user, or their guardian, of this journal.

Remember ~~~ Taking care of YOU is the Best Thing YOU can do for others.

My Medical Manager

For additional copies

https://www.createspace.com/4749039

www.ingramcontent.com/pod-product-compliance
Lightning Source LLC
Chambersburg PA
CBHW070734180526
45167CB00004B/1743